ALL YOU WANTE

The H
Touch
Acupressure

DOLORES RODRIGUEZ

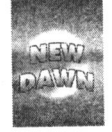

New Dawn

NEW DAWN
a division of Sterling Publishers (P) Ltd.
A-59, Okhla Industrial Area, Phase-II, New Delhi-110020.
Tel: 26387070, 26386209; Fax: 91-11-26383788
E-mail: info@sterlingpublishers.com
www.sterlingpublishers.com

All You Wanted to Know about The Healing Touch (Acupressure)
© 2002, Sterling Publishers Private Limited
ISBN 81 207 2423 2
Reprint 2005, 2007

All rights are reserved. No part of this publication may be reproduced, stored in a retrieval system or transmitted, in any form or by any means, mechanical, photocopying, recording or otherwise, without prior written permission of the publisher.

Published by Sterling Publishers Pvt. Ltd., New Delhi-110020.
Lasertypeset by Vikas Compographics, New Delhi-110020.
Printed at Sterling Publishers (P) Ltd., New Delhi-110020.

Contents

	Gratitude	4
	Preface	5
1.	Touch for Harmony	11
2.	Miracles of Life	32
3.	Vibrating in Harmony	40
4.	Energy Channels	56
5.	Priority Law	114
6.	Energy-Balance	130
7.	Conclusion	151

Gratitude

I want to offer this humble book at the Lotus Feet of Bhagavan Sri Sathya Sai Baba and also to the form of Shirdi Sai Baba. He is more than a Master or a Guru. He teaches us to find the truth, which is health and harmony for every being, through correct action, peace, love and non-violence.

I want to thank Sterling Publishers for this opportunity to share my experience with others. I want to thank their wonderful families for their warm hospitality. I am also grateful to Maria Aragones, the Spanish Publisher, who helped me in my work, to Sean Cook for proofreading the book, and to my family in Spain, who encouraged me to stay in India, and grow in my spiritual work.

Preface

The purpose of this book is to share my experiences on how to acquire a healthy mind and body. I would like to emphasise that this is not a conventional book about acupressure technique. Though I am not a doctor, I have been studying about natural therapies and mind control for more than 15 years. I know that many people need to use conventional medicines and there are many circumstances in which it is necessary. However, I have been looking at an alternate way to deal with illness.

While studying the different natural methods, I have realised the importance of a natural way of life, including spiritual life, studying different spiritual tendencies and different techniques of natural medicine.

I have been studying and practising bioenergy and learning how important it is to channelise energy, especially the universal energy. I also got interested in kinesiology (the study of the mechanics of body movement) during a particularly stressful period in my life. I have studied a complete synthesis of the four most important schools of kinesiology and have investigated the relation and connection between muscles, acupuncture meridians, organs and emotions; and how to get information directly from the brain, through a muscle test, about any circumstance of any health problem. I have also investigated how to resolve problems by using techniques including acupressure points, and electrical, emotional, chemical and structural work. I have also discovered how to programme solutions into the brain so as to affect any new cell in its healing from the beginning. Many psychologists are now interested in this method of healing. It is a good way to obtain directly from the brain any information about traumatic experiences from the past, including pre-birth and how these influence our actual state of health. It also helps to resolve emotional and mental stress that causes health problems. I began to experiment directly with my mind to establish harmony, which helped me to understand, in a scientific way, my previous spiritual work.

After this I experimented with the effectiveness of acupressure points on myself. I could resolve some difficult problems in my body and mind. Then, it was time to learn shiatsu:

a therapy of Japanese origin, in which pressure is applied with the thumbs and palms to certain points of the body.

Their method of working with the acupressure points is not the same. But still it was useful for me to practise and to find the meridian points.

It was also interesting for me, through initiation in reiki, to finally understand how powerful our hands are and how we are a channel of love, of that universal love, which moves everything of which we are a part. Now this has become the most important principle in my life. I know that if we really have this feeling in our lives, we will be healthy and happy beings, full of peace, love and harmony.

Towards the end of the search for integral and holistic harmony, I finally found my way to Bhagavan Sri Sathya Sai Baba. He has been teaching me to differentiate between good and bad qualities in my mind, to be able to open my heart to divine love, and to let this love reach through my life to every being in the universe, because we are all one.

"Om Sai Ram"

Touch for Harmony

I have been experimenting and practising natural therapies of acupressure, kinesiology, shiatsu and reiki on myself and on many people suffering from different diseases under different circumstances. The results have been very good, especially in emotional problems, compulsive behaviour and degenerative problems.

In chronic cases, it is important to identify whether the causes are physical or emotional. If you know and practise these methods on yourself, you will be able to recognise the difference. In order to know all about ourselves and our special needs, like diet, feelings, etc., to pay attention to the small changes taking place in our systems, and to be able to correct them promptly, we need to learn to feel the flow of energy.

This method of learning is a synthesis between kinesiology and shiatsu. While shiatsu takes a better view of meridian points, kinesiology works through a muscle test, which gives and takes information directly from the brain about certain electrical, emotional, chemical and structural circumstances of the patient. This synthesis, must also include some principles of bioenergy and reiki to help correct any malfunction of any part of our system.

About 50 years ago a chiropractor discovered that when he put one hand over any part of the body of a patient, the behaviour of that muscle changed. Through observation it was discovered that muscles are connected with different acupuncture meridians, and that some of them are able to give information about states of energy. Each muscle is also connected to a special area of the brain. It is affected by emotional or mental circumstances in the mind.

Each meridian or electrical point gives energy to certain muscles. When there is stress of any kind, or electrical, emotional, chemical or structural disharmony, it produces a block in energy flow and the power in the muscle goes down.

It is possible to detect this phenomenon through a muscle test. Through this test, a therapist can know exactly what is stressing the particular neurological area and what electrical, emotional, chemical or structural correction is required. It is here that acupressure points are used to correct problems. In our body, stress is engraved in each cell, including that which occured before birth. However priority must be given to resolve the present problems. This is done by asking the brain directly and watching how a stressful matter influences the muscles and acupressure points. Then it is possible to correct this as a priority, using the kind of therapy, that the patient prefers. Every kinesiologist knows how to apply other therapies, like homeopathy, osteopathy, naturopathy, acupuncture or bioenergy, according to the specific needs of the patient.

Coming back to a more scientific point of view, kinesiology is based on a technique of structural function or the relation between face and temper or body and character.

It was a revelation for me to understand the nature of the life of my present body. This technique teaches that the quantity of cells in each part of our face and head, is in the same proportion in each neurologic area of the brain. As each neurologic area is specific to a special function of the body or mind, it is in direct relation to the form of our face, head and body, and also with our temper. We could say that each part of the brain is in some way responsible for one or the other part of our behaviour. The face for example, is a mirror of the mind. This is why we say, "I don't like that face", referring to someone who may be reflecting what we do not like genetically.

We all get an original and unique body which reflects all our mental tendencies. This body is a combination of the images of our father and mother, their ancestors, and all of their character tendencies.

The character of our parents, which is affected by the character of their own parents and so on, also affects us. When we recognise this in our face, or experience it through a traumatic situation, we come to accept that our parents cannot be in another form, nor can they act in a different way. Kinesiology thus is used to resolve the conflict which exists in our minds to accept and recognise our own mental tendencies, or ego, so that we can accept our own features, which also means to accept the character tendencies of our parents, reflected in our own features.

In the same way we are able to differentiate between other people and ourselves, yet know that they cannot be in another form because of their own genes and karma. We are thus able to respect and love them and even understand the law of karma. This is how we can really feel and experience true love in everybody.

It happens, thus, that our character also produces an expression on our face, and this can, over time, produce wrinkles, so that it begins to be marked by time. When we are older our character is already designed on our faces. So a relaxed face is a perfect symbol of inner harmony.

There is another beautiful practice in kinesiology, called pricotherapy, which is said to be a barometer of behaviour. With this technique and through the muscle test, we can find out exactly which emotion or trauma is the cause of any health problem. Then, some very good psychotherapy and energetic exercises can help to free the particular neurologic area, which is affected, as well as the corresponding part in the body, which is in relation with it. These exercises consist of symbols which are visualized in order to liberate the mind of whatever stressful, sad or traumatic memory that is taking the energy from our body.

This is a very good way to liberate oneself from attachment, because all suffering comes from attachment. Suffering produces contraction and sickness. Health problems can be determined depending on the kind of emotion which causes imbalance either on the left or the right side of the body. If it is in the present time, the imbalance is in the front. If it is in the past time, the imbalance is in the back, and so on. It is important to liberate all emotional and mental tension to be truly in harmony.

Suffering is contraction, and faith and love are expansion, health and harmony. [When I found my way to Sai Baba, I also learned a very good method of cutting ties that bind, from Philis Crystal, a very good psychotherapist who lives in America, and travels around the world teaching her methods.] This helped me a lot because it was so similar to what I had been studying. It works in a very simple way, by asking questions directly to our inner being or higher consciousness. Intuitionally, you can know through some very simple but energetic exercises, what exactly is the cause of imbalance or unhappiness and how to resolve it, using visual symbols. Our mind works through symbols. This is similar to the barometer of behaviours. It is not necessary to use the muscle test to ask the mind. We connect with a feeling of faiths, and trust, that our intellect is able to tell us everything about our real nature.

In acupressure, our thoughts influence our energy-balance all the time. When we feel tensed up, our muscles contract and acupressure points become blocked. Energy does not flow. The points become painful. Then, at an energetic point, pressure relieves the pain. This is very natural and instinctive.

In kinesiology it is not possible to experiment on a muscle, if the patient is not feeling the truth. Thus all points in our body are constantly being influenced by our thoughts, our ignorance, our bad tendencies and by external circumstances like diet, temperature, clothes, telluric energies, etc. which are not harmonious. Our energy is moving all the time, and our state is reflected in all our points, and not only in the principal meridian points. Our body has thousands of energetic points. In kinesiology and shiatsu, different pressures are applied to these points.

It is stated in kinesiology that anything can heal anything. Sometimes food can bring about an emotion, and sometimes a positive thought can heal a digestion problem. And so it is with many things. It is necessary to prioritise, and it is possible to use muscle testing, intuition, or to ask our higher consciousness to do this for us. It takes some time and practice to get in touch with our own sensitivity. I shall explain about how to feel energy in the next chapter, through some information about bioenergy.

I also came to know about a very good oriental technique, chibong, which helps clear meridians using movement exercises and postures. As a result you can discover which parts in the body are tense, and help the energy to flow.

When we become sensitive to our energy and pay attention to any change, we can watch the parts in our body that have energy blocks or painful points. By learning about acupressure points and how to find them, we can trust our intuition, and practise asking our higher consciousness, or inner being, to press the points in priority, sending all our tensions and their causes back to the universal energy, which can absorb and transmit them into creative and divine energy.

With practice one can prioritise points. One can say that both horizontal as well as vertical information exist in the body. Horizontal information is that which is obtained through reason, and vertical information comes directly from universal truth. All we have to do is to ask for it, to trust and wait, and it will come. Step by step it becomes natural, and a therapist can come to prioritise directly, after asking a few questions about the circumstances of the patient.

It is also necessary for a patient to understand the cause of each blocked part of the body, while being tested or treated.

There is a sensation when there is anything that makes us unhappy. We are able to feel the most important occurance of the present time. If we continue looking for a more ancient cause when we feel it necessary, this information will come to our conscious awareness from our subconscious mind.

In this way, images will come to our conscious mind from the past into the present. We can recognise them when we press points, using breath (which I shall explain later) to feel the cause of our pain, and knowing that our essential energy is able to dissolve it. Upon sending it to the universal creative energy storage, we feel relaxed in our breath and energy flows again. We can feel electric currents flowing through the meridians. Sometimes we can even feel them from the arm or head, all the way to the foot. It is a great joy. It is the physical, mental and emotional response, which gives us peace, because we are liberating ourselves from mental and physical suffering. The universal energy is transforming it back to its true nature — divine love. Universal energy can appear to us in a concrete form. For, spiritual people, it is possible to choose a special form of divine energy, or any symbol of it. There is a guarantee that this is effective because we are dissolving suffering from our mind and cells, and impressing happiness upon every cell. It is so frequent that people start to cry. This is because of the liberation of old traumas and other blockages.

I shall explain later how to do a therapy session. It is not necessary to do one in a sequential form.

After about three times of applying pressure at each priority point and working with the breath alongside, the pain releases, healing the disease and its cause.

Miracles of Life

A miracle may be defined as anything which is not understood by reason or controlled by the senses or with technical instruments. Today, it is possible to control mental waves through a machine or take a reading of essential energy. Many years ago this would be incredible, like a miracle. Step by step, human beings have been able to comprehend so much more as compared to ancient times. Even now they are discovering new possibilities of being in harmony with the universe.

There are many universal laws which are still not scientifically corroborated, but this does not mean that they do not exist. In my opinion, the greatest miracle in the universe is love — pure love. It is the one true power which is able to move everything. If we really believe this, we can surrender to it and everything will become a miracle in our lives.

Vibration is a miracle. It is also the first sound, 'OM'. Its pronunciation itself is beneficial. Everything in the universe is vibration, alive or inert (from inertia) and existing.

Another miracle is "life" from microscopic to human, which is also vibration. The same vibration is in the microcosmos or macrocosmos, in the sky with its stars and galaxies, or in our body with its cells and microbes.

Chemistry is also a miracle. Everything is controlled in the universe in perfect order. There is a universal force which directs and controls all. And there are many laws which we still do not know. The mind is powerful — creative as well as destructive, and we are completely unaware about how it works. But in an intuitive way we know how great the mind is, and also how powerful the heart is. This is why a very serious illness is sometimes healed spontaneously.

But there are also simple laws which we can experiment with in life to be healthier.

Everything is vibration, and in everything there is polarity, or the *Yin* and *Yang* principle. We are electrical beings, and the current which moves in us is breath. Breath being a part of our vibrating self, is like vibration, a miracle. Life is breath. In the breath are the most important and simple cycles of inhalation and exhalation.

Every being has these two cycles in any kind of breath, in their cells. This is live vibration, and it is very important to become constantly conscious of this fact.

There are many good exercises in bioenergy and kriyayoga for example. Because vital energy is in the air and each ancient culture has this knowledge, we should learn not to waste it at any moment in our lives. So accepting breath as a miracle, it is necessary to learn to breathe completely and consciously, not only using the lungs, but swelling the abdomen area and using and feeling the movement of the diaphragm as well. This is one of the reasons why we should wear comfortable clothes as far as possible. It is very important not to press the thorax and abdomen areas, so that they expand in a free way. In this manner, energy can reach each cell, which will help to bring about a better state of mind. When our lungs are empty, our energy is *Yin*, which comes from the earth and is female. When we inhale, our lungs are full and the energy is *Yang*, which comes from space, and is male. We must observe and enjoy which is the most important circle in life, the manifestation of both parts of divinity — mother and father. If we do this and also practise a healthy kind of life, we become more receptive to feel energized and happy. We are all the time receiving *Yin* energy from the earth and *Yang* energy from the sky, just like a battery. If the battery is loaded, we are full of energy. Then our energetic body becomes great and strong, and we become more sensitive to receiving other energetic stimuli from other people and other things, and we get more information from our own intuition. Energy flows in a better way through our meridians, and our *chakras* become more open and work in a better way. Under these circumstances, meditation is easier, and we can experience the vibration of life in our entire being. We can perceive the pulse, which is life, something like feeling the pulse of our heart in all our being. It in turn produces a vibration which moves our body like a small universe.

Vibrating in Harmony

To experience a balanced mental and physical condition, it is necessary to have a very pure way of life. I would like to discuss here, a little about how to have a more natural and pure life, to be able to vibrate in harmony with the universe.

Talking about breath, we should understand why it is so important to breathe air that is as pure as possible. It is also important in the interest of polarity. Artificial conditions are unhealthy. Artificial materials, in building and decoration or electrical machines which produce ionic unbalance, electro-magnetism, and radioactivity, lead to negative results. Synthetic materials and machines like air-conditioners produce positive ions which are unhealthy, affect the nerves and create stress and tension. It is better to use a fan than an air-conditioner. Plants and natural matter on the other hand, create space with negative ions that are good for health. However, there are also unhealthy agents in nature, for example, telluric lines or subway water.

The mind is very powerful, and if it is really clean, then a miracle is possible. We can be stronger to protect ourselves against unhealthy agents. But this is an extra effort, and as far as possible we must try to live in a natural way. Sometimes we cannot avoid living in a contaminated area, but we can avoid smoking for example, which is so dangerous for our lungs, blood pressure, and other kinds of mental problems.

Since external circumstances affect us, we must be aware of what we wear and what we eat. Nutrition is very important. It is also necessary to be very careful with what our senses absorb, including images, noises and sounds, like television noise or music, whom we touch and so on, because purity is very important. We are working towards being able to work in harmony with energy. If we become very sensitive, more energy transmits through us. We must be a clear channel of purity and love.

It is also important to observe who prepares or touches our food, and where, with whom, when and how we take our food. It is important to take the food always with a thankful and happy feeling. We also need to pay attention to the composition, combination and quality of the food.

Sometimes it is necessary to have a cleansing diet, taking only fruits, and if possible, fasting. It is very good to fast or go on a light diet, particularly when we are very busy or worried. It is also very important at the time of eating to be completely relaxed and feel this time as sacred as possible. Concerning diet, in Ayurveda there is a method of selecting the kinds of food that are good for us, depending on individual temper and constitution.

Circumstances are very important. Activities, including the mind, influence what we need at any moment. (For right thought, it is important that the energy of the food be pure.) There are three kinds of nutrition in Ayurveda: *tamasic* — which stimulates inertia or laziness (*tamas*), *rajasic* — which stimulates passion (*rajas*), and *satvic* — which produces purity (*satva*). We must tend, as much as possible, to the *satvic* state. Everybody should do this, especially those who are interested in energy work. Meat, for example, and food cooked a long time ago are *tamasic*. Food with a strong taste, which is salty or very hot, and stimulating drinks, like coffee and alcohol, are *rajasic*. Vegetables, especially raw or recently cooked and milk and milk products are *satvic*. The combination of each nutrient is also important. It is good to investigate to find out what works for oneself and also the times which are best to eat. Wise people say: eating three times a day means *tamas*. A *yogi* who has only one meal a day experiences that digestion needs a considerable amount of energy. If we save that energy, we can use it for other necessities. We must assimilate nutrients in a better way. Through control of the mind, positive thoughts, and an ordered way of life, prioritising correctly, we can achieve the highest results.

It is recommended to start the day with fruit or some juice to clean our digestive system, and to purify our blood. I insist that one should not eat animal protein. It becomes rotten during digestion, and results in toxicity. Imagine how unwise it is to insert into our body a substance obtained from the suffering of another living being. Vegetables are different, because it has been found that they stay alive till just the moment we need to eat them. This has been measured with scientific apparatus and the results show that their kind of life and frequency of energy is very different from that of animals. It is as if they were created to nourish us.

We must try to be right in every action, and to be in truth with our own nature, which is peace and love. So when people are happy, it is not really necessary to eat so much food. This is why many saints are able to practise what is called *tapas*, because they do not waste any energy at all. They do not repress anything, they need nothing more because they take life's energy directly from its source, through spiritual practices like prayer or meditation.

It is advisable to wear natural and comfortable clothes. It is very important not to press the body in any way, particularly in the areas of the *chakras*. If we cannot breathe in a natural and comfortable way, we may get a headache. This also happens when we wear anything uncomfortable over our head. A funny situation arose when I discovered that in a former life, I was a designer of fashion hats. I used to have a headache whenever I wore one of my more original but uncomfortable hats. At first, I could not figure out why this happened, and why I was not able to enjoy these beautiful moments. Some time later, when I studied bioenergy and kinesiology, I discovered that there are a lot of sensitive points around the head, and that there is something called the craneal breath which consists of a very subtle movement of the cranium bones, and that we must not interfere with it. It is useful not to mark or show as much as possible, the body forms, especially for women. It might evoke feeling and sensitivity when watched by other people and this is no relaxation, but puts more tension and stress on our minds.

There are also some other matters to consider which can help us to be balanced.

Hydration, for example, is very important. Water is one of the most important life-giving forces in the universe. It is also an important part of the body and helps to clean the inside and outside of it. It is necessary to drink as much water as possible to clean our digestive system, to wash our body, to keep everything which belongs to us clean, and to have a more pure life.

Many of us do not know that another reason for drinking water is to ensure electrical balance in our body. Sometimes only a little quantity is enough when we are stressed, nervous, very tired or afraid. Contact with water relaxes us. In these moments it is also very good to urinate because by doing this, we relax muscles throughout the body, and the mind relaxes, too. The toilet and bedroom must be clean, comfortable and as beautiful as possible. They are very important places in our homes. These are the places that we use to clean and take care of our body, and they are symbols for cleaning our being. Dressing our hair liberates us from tension and frees us from attachment to energies from outside.

It is important that clothes should always be clean, but it is also recommendable to change them, especially when we arrive home or do any kind of activity, because clothes get a lot of information and energy from outside activities and it is liberating for us to change them.

It is also important to keep the house in order. It can be simple, and may not be luxurious. Details must be carefully selected and everything should be in its correct place. It must not produce extra stress in us.

There is a study called psychotronic which speaks about materials, colours, forms and some simple techniques to help our brains not to waste energy. It is recommended to keep the temperature of the body as constant as possible. Use of cold or warm water, is called hydrotherapy. We can experiment by observing what our body needs every moment by following our intuition, which is vertical information. It is also very important to observe and to correct our posture and way of walking. While walking, we must pay attention not to waste energy, by concentrating on moving only the essential muscles involved in each movement. Feet must go parallel, arms must not move too much, and the back and head must be upright so that our legs must be supported in a uniform way. We must be calm yet alert and enjoy the whole exercise.

We are really energetic beings, full of pure energy. We are living channels of love, of universal love, which is the duty or dharma of our existence.

Energy Channels

Now it is time to study about acupressure points; how to look for them, and the correct way to apply pressure — that is, where, when and how to press them. To start the treatment there are five factors to be considered:
1. Usual places to find points.
2. Priority law (prioritisation).
3. Ways of applying different kinds of pressure.
4. Ways of breathing during applying pressure.

5. Mental and emotional state at the time of applying pressure.

• Locating the meridians

The first priority is to locate the principal points, which are the meridian points. Meridians are channels of essential energy (Chi O Prana) in the body. It is known that there are *6 pairs of Yin and 6 pairs of Yang (Figures 1 and 2), and two singles* which are located in the central part or the trunk of the body, ascending from the downward area of the trunk to the head. One is in the front part and the other is at the back. The one in the *front* is called the *Conception*

Vessel and finishes just below the inferior lip. That which is at the *back* is called the *Governing Vessel* and ends just above the superior lip.

Three of the Yin meridians ascend from the legs along the *front part* of the body, and *the other three extend from the pectoral area* through the *internal part of the arms and fingers.*

The three which flow from different parts of the foot and toes along the *legs* and ascend to the superior part of the *body* are the *Spleen, Kidney* and *Liver* meridians. The other three which flow along the *interior part of the arms,* are the *Lung* meridian to the thumb, the *Heart* meridian to the nail of the little finger, and the *Heart Constrictor* or *Pericardium* meridian to the middle finger.

There are two kinds of *Yang meridians* also: *three pairs* which *flow down* from the *head* along the *body* and *legs,* and *another three* which flow from the fingers along the *external part* of the *arms to the head.*

Those which flow down along the *body* and *legs* are: the *Stomach* meridian, which is in *front* of the *body* and starts just beneath the eye, in the middle, at the border of the bone which forms the hole of the eye and flows down along the front part of the

Figure 1

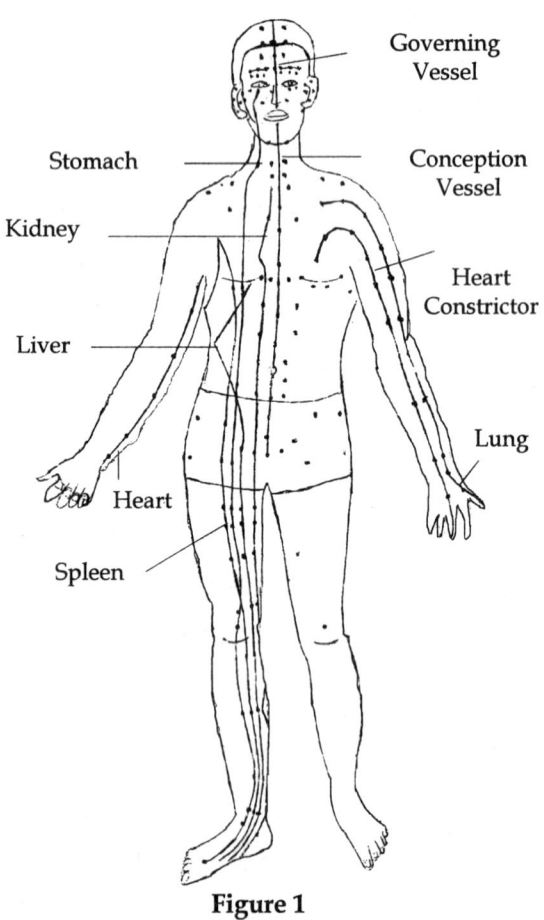

body and the front part of the leg to the foot.

The *Bladder* meridian, which starts at the tear duct and goes up over the head to the *back side* of the head, and after the neck separates into two parts along *the back* to the back part of the knee, down to the small toe in the foot.

The *Gall Bladder* meridian starts from the external part of the border of the hole of the eye, just beneath where the eyebrows finish, and flows down behind the ear along the neck to the shoulder (zig-zags along the *external side of the trunk*) and goes straight along the *external part* of the *leg down* to the small toe.

The *three pairs* which are on the *external part of the arms* (Figure 2) are the *Large Intestine* meridian, travelling from the index finger along the *external part* of the arm and shoulder, neck and face, to the border of the cheek bone.

The *Small Intestine* meridian starts on the nail of the small finger and goes up the back part of the arm over the elbow, to the shoulder and the superior of the back, through the neck to the ear just at the jawbone.

The *Triple Warmer* meridian begins on the nail of the ring finger and continues on the back side of the hand and arm to the shoulder and through the neck, behind the ear, and over to the temple.

Figure 2

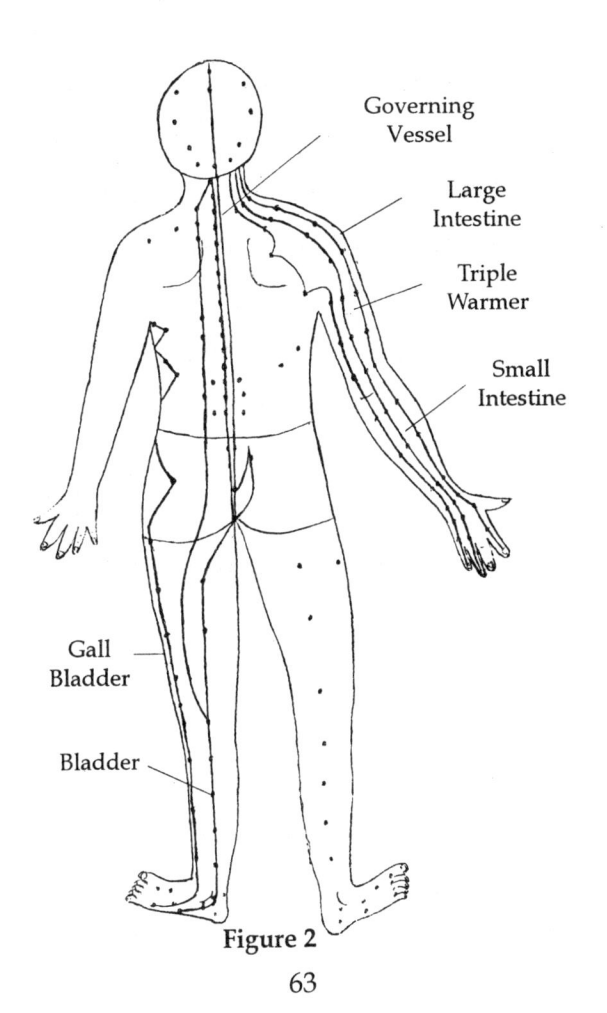

These are the meridians, which are connected with the main organs and systems in the body, and are therefore named after these organs. Each organ receives energy from that respective meridian, and some muscles. One of them in particular is known and used in kinesiology.

There are also subsidiary meridians. Special points of the meridians are studied to heal different problems. There are actually many thousands of points, and we can discover what is necessary for each of them.

Each meridian has 24 hours in a day and only one moment of maximum energy and one moment of minimum energy. This takes place during a two hour period. After the maximum moment, the energy passes to the next meridian in the energy circle. There is a wheel which is divided in twelve parts of 2 hours each for any one meridian. For example, energy flows starting from the liver at 1 a.m. to the lungs, large intestine, stomach, spleen, heart, small intestine, bladder, kidney, pericardium, triple warmer and finally to the gall bladder from 11 p.m. to 1 a.m. (Figure 3).

In this way, when one of them is in maximum energy, the opposite is at its minimum. For example, if the maximum period of energy for the lungs is from 3 to 5 a.m., at the same time, the meridian which is opposite, i.e. the bladder is in a period of minimum energy. And so it goes along each 24 hours. So, whenever

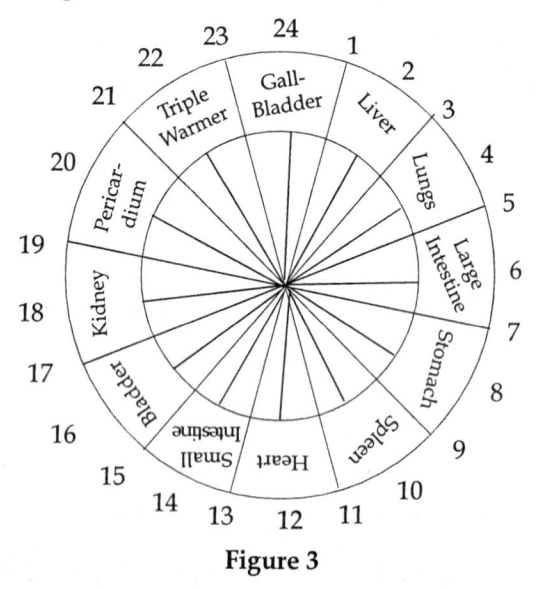

Figure 3

there is a block because of mental or physical cause, energy does not flow correctly. One meridian flows in excess, keeping a lot of energy, and the other especially the opposite one, flows too little. Thus there is an imbalance, and when there is an imbalance, there is a problem which is necessary to correct.

For good results, it is important to be careful with any part of the body which is injured or scarred. It is possible to help these areas by applying energy lovingly with the hand, like in the reiki system, after working the adjacent areas.

Locating the pressure points

Our bodies are covered with pressure points. Different points are to be treated differently. Certain points can be found by observing where the energy is circulating.

It is possible, for example, to find points at the central parts of muscles, on the head of the bone in an articulation, at the borders of big bones, and over the bones themselves.

Starting on the head, there are points of different meridians, as mentioned earlier in the chapter, through the cranium, face and around the ears and neck.

The pressure points of the governing vessel, at the central area of the bladder, are *through the cranium*.

The pressure points for the small intestine, triple warmer, and gall bladder meridians are *around the ears*.

On the face are the governing vessel meridian, conception vessel, large intestine meridian, stomach, bladder, triple warmer meridian and gall bladder meridian.

Through the neck passes the governing and conception vessel, and all the yang meridians. These are the stomach, in front of the body, the bladder, at the back, and the gall bladder, at the side. The yang which flows through the external parts of the arms are the large intestine, small intestine, and triple warmer, meridians.

We know that there are other subsidiary meridians, which can help find some other useful points, in certain places. Some of them are shown in figures 4 and 5, respectively. Similarly, in kinesiology, there are some very useful points at the *corners of the cranium* that are called *neurovasculars*, because they provide energy to the blood and circulatory system for the brain. When any area of the brain is under stress or very tired, these points cannot work as they are supposed to. As a result blood is not provided in correct quantity to that particular area. This gives rise to a health problem, because everything in our system is in direct correlation with a neurologic function. By pressing these points, it is possible to help them, through a massage, to work correctly again. Usually it is better to press softly to relax them, especially if the points are very painful. But at other times there are some points which should be pressed with more strength, paying attention to the breath, to quickly resolve the problem.

Next to the ears there are pressure points everywhere—just in front of the hole, at the superior and inferior borders, over the bone at the back area, all around the ear, and inside as well. These points are very small and painful. There are so many points in the body which can be pressed with the kunckles and, of course, with the finger, but around the ear, it is better to use something like a nail or other pointed object. It is only on the ear proper and not around it, which is to be pressed with the fingers.

On the face there are three very important points over the forehead as we can see in Figure 4. One is in the middle, and the other two on both sides (1, 2, 3). There is a very good technique to relax the mind using this area. There are points over the eyebrows (4, 6), generally at the borders of the bones, and in the middle and between them. The last one is a very important point for stimulating the third eye *chakra* (5).

Under the eyebrows, at the soft part between the bone of the eyebrow and the eye, there are some points to release stress (Figure 4). There is also one point situated in this area which is very good for nose discomforts or colds. It is close to the nose, just like the ones over the eyebrows. There is

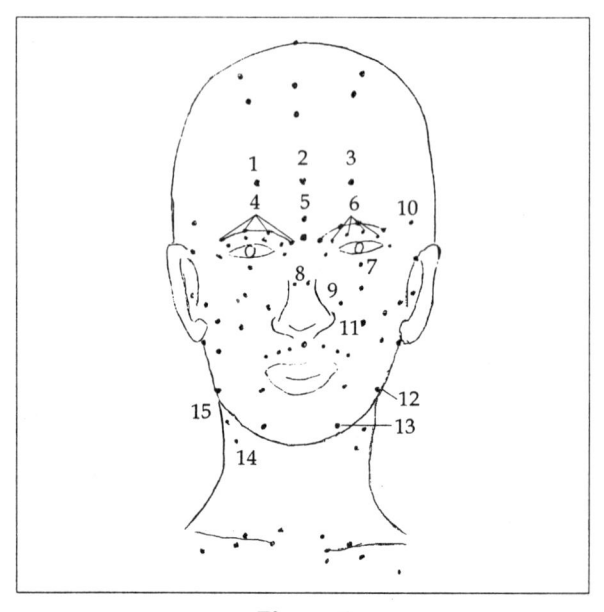

Figure 4

one point under the eye, which is the first point of the stomach (7) and over the nose bone (8). There are also points on both sides of the nose (9), at the temple (10), and under the cheek bone (11). Depending on the cause of a cold or location of pain, on congestion, points of pressure need to be corked on following the law of priority. There is also one very important point for stress release at the end of the jawbone (12), and two others at the border of both sides of the chin bone (13 and 14). Where there is a border of a bone, or a hole between them, it is easy to find a painful point.

For the face, it is important to know that over the teeth, where each one originates, is a point which helps a lot when the tooth is in any problem, as in an infection. (16, 17, 18) (Figure 5).

Many nerves pass over these points, and they can be helped in the

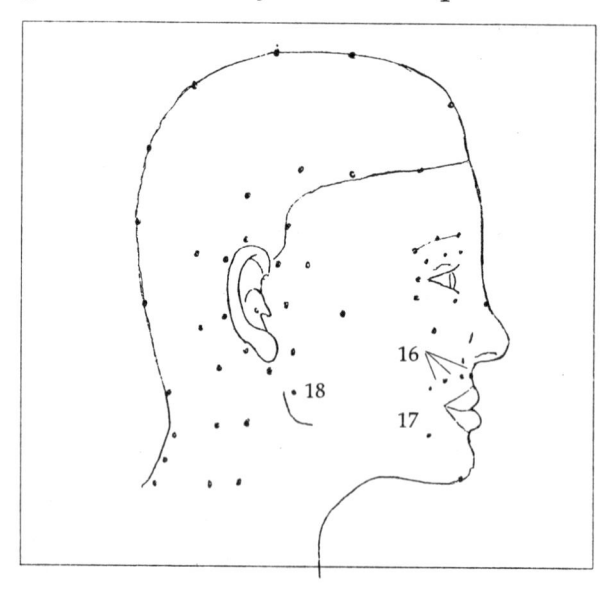

Figure 5

case of neurologic pain by massaging them. One of these points helped me a lot when I had 'zoster herpes' on my cheek. I did not know why a point under my mouth relieved my great pain. Later I discovered that the trigeminus nerve passes directly over that point, and that it was responsible for my pain.

The points of the neck are in special relation with the different parts of the head.

There are some very useful points for stress, gripe and colds, just under the occiput or base of the skull, as well as along both sides of the cervical vertebra.

At the front part of the neck there are some points on both sides under the chin and jawbone that are in relation with the ganglions (14, 15) (Figure 4). They must be massaged very carefully. The points on both sides of the larynx can also help resolve throat disease. It is necessary to look very carefully at a very small painful point and to keep pressing it softly.

At the front part of the body, over and under the clavicle, there are some very uncomfortable points which are painful in an electrical way, that can be massaged by barely touching them. It is a very uncomfortable sensation, but it is very good for electric and polarity imbalance. This is usually produced after a very busy journey to artificial places like airports, supermarkets or shopping malls, and if we are speaking to different people about different matters. This area is also very useful for the immune system, as is the highest part of the sternum, where the thymus gland is situated. It is very good to hit this area with the fist several times, and also the spleen area (just on the left side over the border of the rib cage beneath the pectoral area), where there is a point which affects the spleen function responsible for renewing red blood cells. If it does not do its job properly, anemia may result. The thymus is a gland whose size depends on the quantity of our happiness. That is why its growth is stopped at an early time in our life, when the inner happiness, which is our real nature, is overshadowed by worldly matters. This is also why we become old.

It helps us stimulate these areas by hitting them frequently, like big gorillas do. In kinesiology it is good to do it 21 times a day. It is also very important to have in our mind an image or a mantra which produces in us as much happiness as possible.

This helps our immune system prevent and heal infections.

Continuing through the body, there are some very important points in the *front of the pectoral area between the ribs*. Sometimes it is very good to rub these in a transversal way, along the ribs. This is also very uncomfortable, just like the clavicle part, but it gives great results, and after massage comes an incredibly relaxing sensation. It is possible then to feel that energy is flowing through the whole area.

A very important point about these points of T is how they can help women with mammary gland problems. I could avoid surgery two times during a particularly stressful time in my life. It gives a real feeling of liberation from other emotional pains that women often have, especially in relationships. It happens that with this kind of frustration, hormonal imbalance is created and energy is blocked in these points. There is a contraction of texture around the blocked points. Expansion is happiness and contraction is sickness. The contraction starts a degenerative process and it is necessary to stop it as soon as possible. This kind of massage helps to dissolve this destructive process.

When energy flows again, the texture becomes more distended. The flow of energy helps to restore hormonal balance, and the way to emotional resolution reopens.

Often the *heart chakra* is also in contraction, and we make ourselves weak and frail. But there is a technique which can be applied to reduce heart contraction. It is not a simple technique, because this pressure point is a very soft and delicate one. It is located at the hole under the sternum. We must press the point with the three principal fingers, slowly, and with the lungs empty. It is very important to do this correctly, exhaling slowly and keeping slight pressure until we can support it as comfortably as possible. Then there will be a specific pain, like sadness of the heart. It is even more important to try to understand the emotional cause of this pain. After some time inhale again in a natural manner, enjoying it as much as possible, and liberating negative emotion every time you exhale.

After at least three times, change the process, and inhale as much as possible, trying to open the heart, with hands over the ribs on both sides of the hole as if trying to open them. At this moment, divine energy will flow, liberating all tensions. This work is also possible in the solar plexus and navel area. *At the navel*, it is little different, because it is very important not to press directly over the navel. There are eight points around it, like a cross, and another between it, like an eight pointed star. As we try to find which of these points are painful, we should be *working to the right, very carefully* because the pain can be very uncomfortable, as if the sense of existence is in contraction. Press softly with the lungs empty till the painful area is found, always turning to the right. Do a circle more to find the exact point of most pain and press a little more step by step. The patient will exhale as pressure is applied to each point, and at the end of every circle he can rest and breathe naturally. It is very important to start always from the superior part, at the point just above the navel, and find the most painful point. Repeat pressure, making it a little stronger each time to relieve the pain. It is possible to liberate tension with this technique, and of course the associated emotion as well. When pressing, feel the pain of life, and afterwards, when the pain is relieved, inhale a lot, inflating the entire abdomen area and keeping as much air in as possible, to feel the divine energy of life. Repeat this several times and then rest and enjoy the new status of liberation that follows. Causes of problems in the front part of the body, are usually mental or emotional circumstances in the present time.

Continuing with the points at the front part of the body, we find some at the *lower part of the abdomen*, on a vertical line on both sides under the navel, which help women during menstruation problems or kidney pain. There are also points that are very good for women, over the pelvis, just at the border of the iliac and also under it, in the hole. Others are at the articulation of the leg and the connection of the femur and pelvis. These are very good points to press by rubbing in a transversal way for uncomfortable pain. Lastly, over the pubic bone, there are points which help to overcome any problem or congestion of the sexual and reproductive organs, both male and female, and which also helps women during menopause. These points are very helpful in case of electrical imbalance, which produces other kinds of diseases which affect concentration and mental work, like different dislexias and imbalance in perception.

Some of these points are used in kinesiology neurolymphatics because they provide energy to the lymphatic system, and some of them are connected directly with the ganglions, and help to resolve many different kinds of problems. Some of these points are massageable.

As I said before, the body is full of points, almost everywhere there is some kind of point. But there are also some that are used more frequently. For example, those which are *on both sides of the vertebrating spine*. There are two lines of bladder meridian whose points are connected to different functions, organs and parts of the body, depending on how high the point is situated in relation with a superior or inferior area.

The points on the superior part or dorsal part of the body should be used for stress. Neck points help in throat, sinus infections and cold. The entire thoracic area is recommended for these kinds of diseases, as also points on the shoulder (over or near the shoulder blade) and some points in the middle of the arms and hands. Those along the dorsal part of the spine reflect a more physical tiredness. They also affect functions and organs which are situated at the superior part of the abdomen, like the digestive organs, pancreas, spleen, and diaphragm. Basically at the lumbar area, points indicate functions and organs of the lower part of the abdomen, like the kidneys, both intestines, sexual and reproductive organs, legs, feet, and other organs in the (lower) parts of the body. All these points are useful for any kind of problem regarding bones, blood, muscles and their functions, depending on which area is interrelated with the particular point.

Concerning the *sacrum area*, there are points on both sides adjacent to the border of the sacrum bone, which can be massaged. One may also apply pressure in small circles in one direction depending on the feeling of the patient. Just over the bone, there are four pairs of points, which we can press in a simple way. This helps a lot with sexual organs and diseases in relation to them.

Problems reflected on the back side generally has a cause in the past. By correcting it in the present time we can heal memories of trauma which are in our subconcious mind. Finally, the *trunk of the body* has a point just under the cocyx, which the patient himself should massage directly. It is better not to intimidate a person, especially if he is of the opposite sex. It is easier for a person himself to feel and apply the exact pressure which is necessary. It is necessary to do this carefully, and to keep one's breathing normal to help dissolve tension and to relax. Sometimes it is necessary to calm the area. Usually in one session it is possible to calm many points after a few applications of pressure to the cocyx area. This point is in direct relation with polarity imbalance in the male and female energy, and it can help homosexual people who sometimes are in confusion about their energy. They may need some kind of stimulation in this area. The point also relates to energy imbalance in the excretory *chakra*.

Legs are instruments for walking, so any discomfort in this area reflects a disposition or circumstance of not being able to move forward. We know, now, that six meridians flow through this area, four at the front part (stomach, liver, spleen and kidney), one at the back side (bladder), and one more at the external side (gall bladder).

It is not necessary to know the particular anatomical names. We only need to look for points. That is, we look for points just over the muscles, at the borders of them, and just over and next to the bones where there is something like a special kind of hole along the bone. While practising, it is easy to find them. People become sensitive and frequently put their finger directly over the painful point. It is necessary to have trust. Texture on these points are a little different, a little more soft. The texture does not present as much resistance to pressure as other parts.

There is a unit to measure distance between points which is equal to the width of the thumb. There is no other way to measure this distance other than to be sure where to place the finger. On the legs, for example, it is possible to find the most important points on each line from the highest part of the thigh, through the middle part, and down to the lower part of the thigh before the knee area with the help of the unit. The same applies to the knee, around it, and the external and back side. Only at the back of the knee it is not good to press over the articulation, but on points above and below it. Painful points along one meridian line gives a better idea of which places they usually are in and experience will show you how to touch them.

In the lower part of the legs, you must follow the central part of the tibia bone from below the knee, while in the middle part and down to the area just before the articulation of the foot, be very careful not to press over sinew areas, at places of articulation.

The external side of the leg is connected to the gall bladder meridian. On both sides of the lower part of the leg, about four fingers over the ankle, there is a very good point for menstruation problems.

Coming to the hands and feet there is an interesting reflexology activity which is explained later. I am including two drawings with information about reflexology from the book, *Be your own doctor* by Dr. Dhiren Gala. Figures 6 and 7.

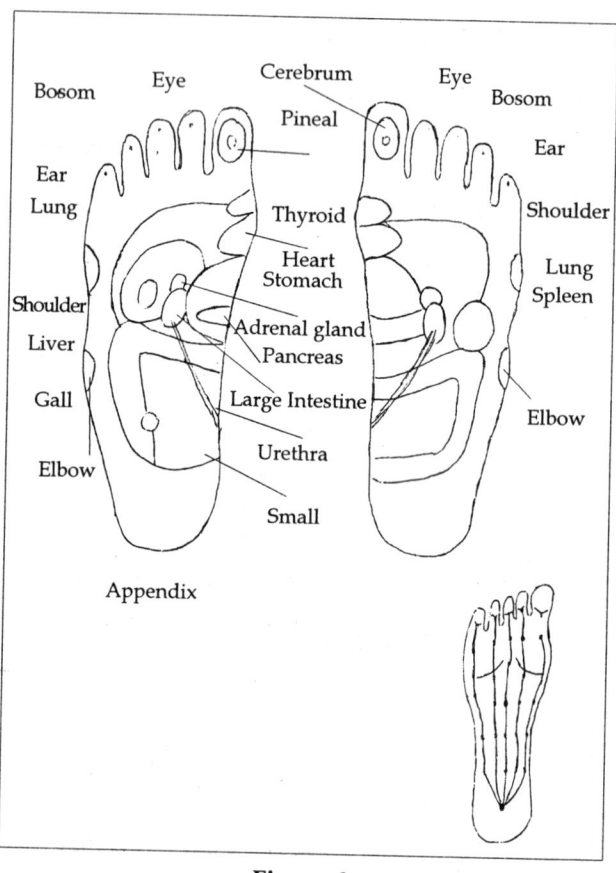

Figure 6

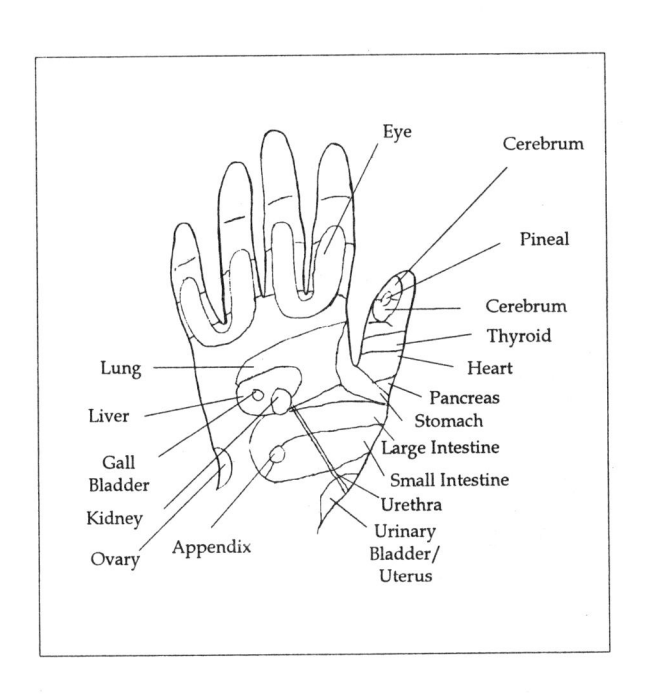

Figure 7

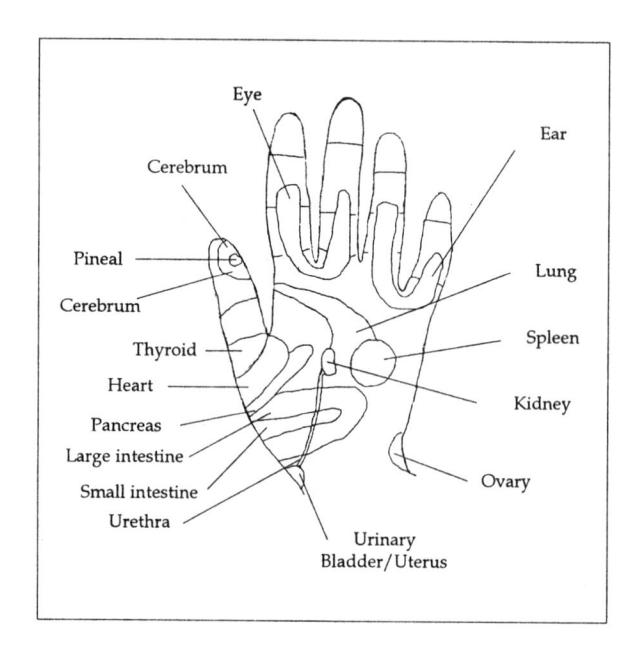

Figure 8

Reflexology connects us with mother earth, and our body is reflected on them.

Referring to acupressure the centre of the body is completely covered with points. It is very good to touch and experiment by applying pressure to any painful point and to the points at the beginning or end of meridians.

Since the foot does not have a big surface, it is good to test for painful points along its entire area. If not many points are painful, it is only necessary to press those which are in priority. Sometimes, when it is not possible to test for painful points on the whole body, it is recommended to work only on the points of the feet and hands or face that are the most painful points to correct any general imbalance.

At the *superior part of the foot* (Figure 6), find the first point at the end of the tibia bone, just in the articulation, and the other three points further down. Then test along parallel lines at both sides of this central line, paying attention as usual to the typical places between bones on the small holes.

There are some points at the ankle bone on both the external and internal parts. One is just above the bone and the other around it, down midway between the ankle bone and the furthest point of the heel.

Just at the bottom of the heel, at the base of the Achilles bone, there is another important and painful point for intestines, rectum, anus and tumors.

Continuing the external line along the base of the foot, there are four points which are very useful for diseases, infections, and general cleansing. On the inner border of the foot, these points correspond to the spine.

Referring to *the toes*, there are three points over each of them, one over each small bone (phalange), and one on both sides of the nails and at the corners between each toe.

There are also points at the union between the toe and the foot, at the small middle articulation, and at the middle of the tips of the toes as well.

Finally, *on the sole* there are five lines which start on a very important point just in the middle of the base of the heel. There are five points on each line along the sole. One very important and particularly painful point is in the middle of the foot, which is the first point of the *Kidney* meridian. There is another just over, between and around the two prominent round structures which look like two balls.

Let us look at the points along the *arms*. We already know that there are 6 meridians flowing along the arms. Three *Yin* flowing from the pectoral area to the fingers along the inner part of the arm, which are — the lung meridian at the most external part, the heart constrictor or pericardium at the middle part, and the heart at the innermost part. Their work is similar to the legs. It is necessary to start from the uppermost part and proceed down, but I usually do both sides of the arm first, and then the hand.

Let us look at Figures 1 and 2 (pgs. 60 & 63) and start working through each of the three inner lines. The lung line starts at the inner part of the shoulder, at the inner border of the head of the humerus bone. Another line begins just at the front part of the head of the humerus, and the next just at the border below it. Next come the points at the end of the shoulder, at the middle part of the arm just before and after the front part of the elbow, at the middle part of the forearm, two over the wrists, and one more just at the union between the arm and hand on the wrist. There is also one very important and painful point on the hand, just over the soft part before the thumb.

The next meridian, the heart constrictor or pericardium, starts on the nipple and ascends to the shoulder. Another point is in front of the armpit, and all succeeding points are at the same height of the lung meridian. However, there is one very important point directly in the middle of the palm.

On the heart meridian, next to the inner part of the arm, there are some points from the armpit to the hand which finish at the small finger, running to the external part just over the nail. The *Yang* meridians are at the back of the arm. I recommend working the most superior points when working on the back of the points along the superior part of the spine and the other points after the front part of the trunk. The principal points are under the shoulder, in the middle of the arm and just before and after the elbow. At the middle of the forearm, just at the wrist, and just after it over the external part of the hand, are the lines which go to the index finger (for the large intestine), the ring finger (for the triple warmer), and the small finger (for the small intestine).

The *hands* are similar to the feet, they reflect everything and it is possible to work more intensively with them. We can find other pressure points on the meridians (Figures. 7 & 8 from pgs. 99 and 100). If you look at Figures 9 and 10, you have an idea of how to work the hands. Besides the arms, head and body, there are many priorty points. Energy blocks are dissolved, and the flow is re-established again and painful points, are reduced. When you cannot have a full therapy session, discomfort or disease may increase and some are really painful. Hence, you must create a balance. It is very convenient to massage by pressing the hands anytime anywhere and it is a very good method to create a balance. It is effective because when there are blocks in the body they are also there in the hands, and if you dissolve these, those which are in the body are released.

The points on the hands are very painful when you are not used to working them frequently, but they get better when you begin to press them. Often, only a moment after applying pressure is the pain relieved.

To practise how to find many points on the hands, it is best to first test the back of the hand and afterwards the palm.

If we look at Figure 9, we can see the points along the external part. It

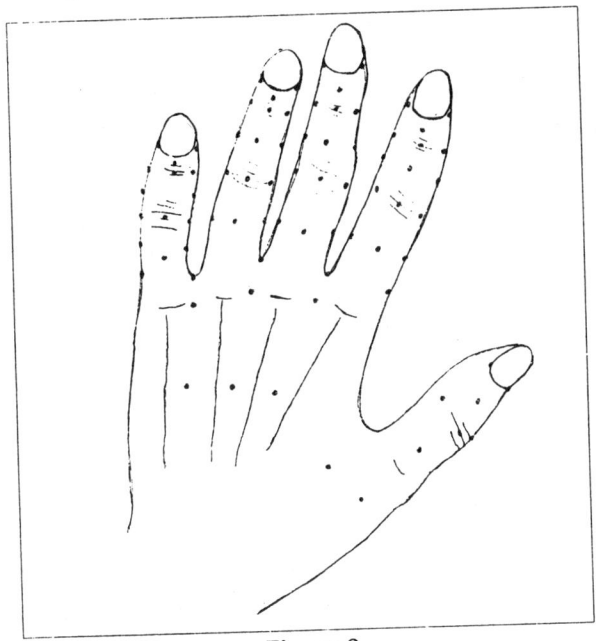

Figure 9

is not necessary to explain each one of them, because it is easy to practise if you observe where they are situated. I find it better to begin with the superior part and continue towards the fingers. Priority points

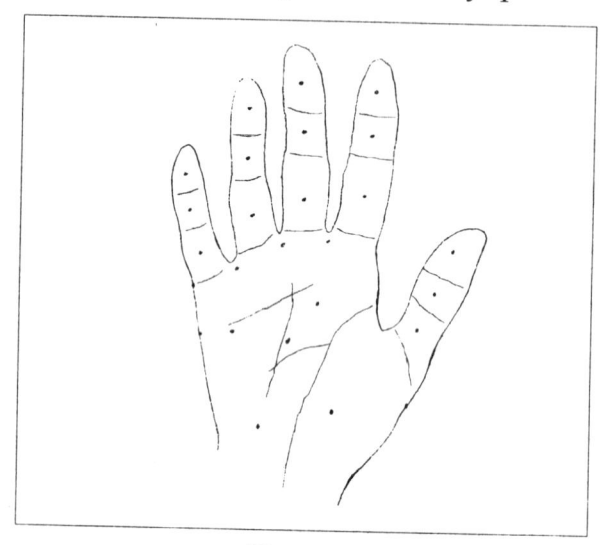

Figure 10

are usually at the more central parts in the body and if correct energy begins to flow to periphery areas, then it can continue in a sweeping fashion to these parts, to rectify them. It is the same along the interior part of the hand or palm, which can be seen in Figure 10.

Priority Law

There is always something which demands most of our attention in the present time, and, of course, takes a big part of our energy as well. It takes energy from different areas of our brain and meridians. It may be a discomfort or disease or function in a particular area of our body or mind.

Usually, this situation arises because of a special debility or trauma circumstance in the past, which is re-occuring and continuing in this way throughout our life. I believe that this depends on the individual work, on the *karma* of each person.

There is always a priority matter in the present time. If you work enough on your mind, and help the memory cell through applying pressure to points, it is possible to clean the mind of conscious and subconcious memories that are taking away most of our energy. Thereafter our energy flows and can be used in a positive way to work good in the world.

During a therapy session go directly to the most contracted and blocked area. It is very useful to practise stretching exercises like Quigong. It is recommended to start from the head, because the machine of all our mental work is our brain. The face is like the mirror of our mind. If we relax and correct all our head and face tensions and blocks, then it is necessary only to clean and correct the effects produced and reflected on different parts of the body. Psychotherapy and energetic exercises liberate the emotional and mental stress.

• **The order to follow in a therapy session**

Though we know that the principal problem is in a concrete area, it is good to have an order to work the different parts of the body. I usually work the back after the head and face, because the back is the most important part where mental and physical work is reflected. It is through the spine that our body receives information from the brain. Our body is a reflection of our mind. It is good to continue with the back part of the legs, then turn the patient over and work the front part of the trunk, which provides energy to organs and functions more in relation with chemical work in the body and the emotions which are in direct relation to it. This also includes hormones and other organic fluids like bile, gastric fluids, insulin, etc.

Finally, we do the front part of the legs, and in the end, the feet. It is very good to finish with the feet, as it completely relaxes the person.

It is very good to learn about the points in the central part of the body, because the blocks are pushed to periphery areas when we finish liberating them and then outside of our being to eliminate any energy block or tension.

The next important factor in the priority law is to know which parts really need to be worked on and which points only need the pressure application.

This work is not really sequential like in shiatsu massage, but it is good to follow an order. It is not really necessary to apply pressure to every point on every meridian. You can test which parts are in contraction and which points are painful and work specifically with them. It is not necessary to press all the points with the same attention and intensity, nor to do both sides in exactly the same way. It does not need to be a bilateral work because both the hemispheres or sides of the brain are not normally working together and in the same way in each person. This is why problems and imbalance in male and female energy occur. It is the same for the front and back. The front relates to concentration and creativity conciousness associated with the thought of work, and the back part, or hypothalamus area, helps us to work and gives a feeling of protection. It is here that fear is registered from every traumatic memory from the past. In kinesiology it is called the "integration common area". It is more extensive work, and very useful for stress. If you press only the priority points, energy flows again. Other points which are painful also heals, after pressing on them in a way which is more intense according to their priority. This does not mean you must press very strongly on the more painful points.

Energy flows and moves through the meridians and sub-meridians along the parts of the body (like cramps) usually all the way to the hands and feet. If the patient pays enough attention and becomes more sensitive, it is possible, especially when he is working with himself directly, to feel very small electrical pricks at the next points to be worked on. This is not always the next point on the meridian nor at the same part of the body. If you press a priority point, properly along the pectoral area often enough, you will feel small electrical pricks in different parts of the body, sometimes even on the other side of the body. That should be the next point to press because energy flows very quickly when a priority point is resolved. Energy quickly arrives to the next block. This method is very good because it goes directly to the causes of discomfort in a rapid way. This is because energy does not think, it flows, and our brain does not give us information consciously through reason only, but also in a subsconscious and indirect way.

There are points other than meridian points. This means that you can find a painful point anywhere. Depending on what quality it is, it is necessary to apply different kinds of pressures.

• Ways to apply pressure

The points of contraction are released through *massage,* using our fingertips. Our nails should be neither too short nor too long. We should use the fingertips for the most delicate areas, like the spaces between the eyes and eyebrows, some points on the head, and any place we need to press more carefully. Sometimes it depends on the nature of the pain and the feeling of the patient to support a stronger pressure. If the breath is under control, then it is possible to press more strongly and frequently, and the pain relieves more rapidly. In this case, it is good to use the knuckles of the index finger and thumb. This is also good for very strong people or people with big muscles or with harder surfaces in the body under points.

There are other ways to apply pressure at the neurolymphatic points, for example between the ribs, and thigh, at the articulation area, the external side and on the *gall bladder* meridian. This is done by rubbing with the tips of three or four fingers, three or four knuckles, or with the external border of the hand.

Finally, there are some very small points to be pressed with any kind of *pricking object*. There is one, which is used professionally, called a *Jimmy*. Sometimes a nail or the blunt end of a pencil or something similar can be used to press some points at the ears, head, hands or feet. These act as if they are situated at the most superficial part of the skin. It is not really necessary to press them strongly, but to apply the force on a very small surface.

I have heard about some shiatsu masters who do not need to press any points. They simply concentrate all their attention and energy on them. This is a very heightened state of conciousness, but we can attempt to experience it when we become highly sensitive to energy and receptive to the minimum imbalance which is produced.

Breathing

This is not shiatsu massage, though the principle of energy is the same in all therapies. Breath is used in a similar way as it is used in bioenergy exercises, that is, by keeping it inside the lungs during the moment of pressure. Not with the lungs completely full or empty, but with a comfortable feeling. Now and again, the patient can do as he feels most comfortable with. But normally it is better to keep some quantity of air inside to send the essential energy to the blocked point. The blocks are released suddenly with an electric effect and you feel relaxed. Just after the pressure it is very good to relax and exhale as much as possible and to keep the hand of the therapist over the point to dissolve the tension completely. If this is done several times on every priority point, it will dissolve energy blocks, congestion and tension.

Mental and emotional work at the time of applying pressure is also very important. Normally when a person has discomfort or disease, he is very stressful and it takes a lot of energy out of him, and he tries to find out the priority to resolve it. One must have trust and be totally sure that the body and mind can be restored through the treatment. The stressful matter may disappear. This does not mean that there does not exist difficulties in life when you practise this treatment. However, it does mean that you will develop enough capacity to overcome them. The mind and the intellect will help to resolve them. It is possible, step by step, to maintain low levels of stress. This is called detachment. So, after discovering what the principal cause of your unhappiness is, try to be receptive to images that may come to your mind during each moment of applying pressure. Then, when you keep the breath inside the lungs, feel and really believe that divine energy is in you, as this will help you. After the pressure is applied on each point, when you exhale, send all your tensions and sufferings to the universal energy to transmit it to positive energy. During the relaxed moments of therapy, after each pressing, relax and calm the texture, and enjoy the moment completely, like a feeling of total happiness, as in reiki therapy.

Energy-Balance

In acupuncture, it is possible, with needles, to help the energy to flow correctly and to establish balance again. The same is true with acupressure.

Sometimes it is necessary to stimulate the points of a meridian which is low in energy, and other times it is necessary to relax those which are in excess. This is possible by using, different forms of pressures, like making very small circles with the finger on the right to create more energy and to the left to create less energy.

How can we know which is necessary? In acupuncture there is a lot of information about what is necessary for a particular circumstance. In shiatsu massage, it is possible to know, depending on the state of the point to be pressed. If it is in contraction and is in excess or is soft and our finger sinks upon pressing it, then it is in low energy, and it is good to press doing the small circles to the right. But I have also experienced, that it is possible to know by simply feeling what is more comfortable to us and what gives us more comfort. Through practice and intuition, we can acquire more sensitivity to these kinds of feelings which are not really difficult, and can be very effective. It helps to choose a good moment to do a therapy session. How to choose the points most necessary, and the way to use the breath to work with them will be explained later.

It is important to know that this treatment is free from harmful side-effects, although, sometimes it is possible to suffer some discomfort because the body is purifying. When energy moves, many changes are produced in the body and the mind. Energy affects emotions, and emotions are chemical, so they, in turn, affect the hormonal system, putting many things in movement to heal. All these changes can produce in us a kind of discomfort. But do not worry because of this. Be positive and receptive to any change in your life's circumstances, physical or mental which could lead you to better health.

Knowing when to practise the therapy comes with practice.

I have experienced, for example, that for back pain it is not very good to get up from bed in a hurry. It is good to press both sides of the spine, putting our knuckles just under the back at the painful points where they are pressed by the weight of the body. This moment is very good because the body is relaxed. It is even better if we freshen ourselves and drink a little water before a session. It is not recommended to have a session after a hot bath. It is also a very good way to start the day, and it helps us to feel stronger and happier throughout the day, especially if we attend to our mental, emotional and spiritual feelings during this process. If we practise this sincerely, our systems will be cleaner and work better. As we clean and nourish our bodies daily, we should also ensure that our energy is kept in balance. Otherwise it takes longer and the pressure points become more painful. But all this depends on the circumstances of the mind. In a really happy being, it is not necessary to do any work, only to enjoy, to be alive in a harmonious body.

In acupressure there are special moments to enjoy the therapy, i.e. when the person is alone, and when he is in a good disposition to work on himself.

At other times of treatment, it is better to be in a relaxed state, not to be under stress, and to be comfortable. It is best to be neither hungry, nor to have your stomach full. It is important also to have the treatment in a clean, quiet and healthy place, with good energy, which is as neutral and natural as possible.

During a session a patient can move or change his posture if he needs to, at any time, because this helps the energy to flow, which in turn helps to feel the next point to press, or the next part in contraction. This is done according to the priority law, where you do not need to follow the typical order of points to press.

The patient should put his hand over any part of the body during the session. The order of areas to work on each part of the body during a session is as follows:

To begin with, it is necessary that both the patient and the therapist feel comfortable. The patient should be straight with his arms and legs parallel, and the therapist should sit behind his head. The therapist should assume a position that will calm his mind. That is, one hand over the forehead and the other one just behind the nape of his neck. This is very good for stress because the energy flows from the back (defence) to the front (creative), and balance is restored. Another kinesiology technique is to put the three tips of the principal fingers from both hands on the two vertical lines just over the eyes and keep the pressure until the pulse is felt. Normally it is not at the same time on both sides because the activity on both the right and left parts of the brain are not in balance. So, during a moment of quiet breath, the therapist should simultaneously finish pressure to restore balance. It is therefore very important that the mind of the therapist be quiet, or he will influence the patient. It is also very good to press the points which correspond to the third eye, to stimulate it to open, which is very useful for concentration. We test and press points on the eyebrows, temple, and the area beneath the eyebrows at the hole between the bone and the eye. By doing this carefully, we can find a particularly hard and painful texture which are very small muscles to move the eyes. This helps to provide us enough energy to work on any particular matter. In kinesiology this is called positive emotional charge. Then we press beneath the eyes, which is the first point of the stomach, then the nose, cheek, and other points of the face, ears (both around and inside), and finally on the head from up the back part at both sides to the nape of the neck. Then we press the neck and continue with the back points with the therapist at the side of the patient. It is good to first do a mild test on points on both sides of the spine to know which part is blocked, and then to go from top to bottom through the points we have studied, paying attention to the priority law. It is good to press first the part nearest to the spine and then to continue through the most external parts, from top to bottom and from shoulder to lumbar through the pelvic area.

There is a technique which can help to correct structural problems of the nortabra and spine, which consists of massaging softly between the fixed vertebra. For rotation, always press softly on the healthy part, and very carefully massage the damaged and painful part. Then press the healthy part again. This helps to stimulate the natural process of correction and if the energetic causes are also corrected at the same time, the problem will be spontaneously resolved.

To continue, we shall press the points on the back part of the legs, then the front part of the body from top to bottom, down to the pelvic area, and out to the arms, hands and the front part of the legs. Finally, we finish with the feet.

In order to become conscious about our inner capacity to heal, it is advisable that we know a little about some energetic qualities with regard to the hands. Currently, the hands are accepted as a part of our body which reflects all our organs and functions. The same is with the feet. This is called reflexology.

Reflexology is different from acupressure treatment. Acupressure is based on correcting the imbalance which produces the disease. In reflexology, massage produces electrical waves that bring the organ back to health. It stimulates the organ or function in a different way, to affect it indirectly. It acts like a mirror which sends the organ information to heal and calm.

So reflexology massage is different from acupressure massage because the form used to press is not the same. But I must say that I am not a reflexologist, so I cannot explain it in a deep way, and that this is not a reflexology book. However, it might be useful to know some reflexology points on the hands and feet (see Figures 6 and 7).

Additional information which is in alignment with this work is from

Ayurveda, and from ancient cultures like the Chinese, which explain the different kinds of energy for each finger in respect to the qualities of the five elements: earth, fire, water, air and ether.

We are composed of these five elements, like everything in material creation. Each of these provides us a special energetic quality necessary to live in a body.

In this way, the different qualities are related to various functions, organs, behaviour and character, as well as nutrients and natural agents which affect us every moment.

Energy is in movement all the time. We need to connect with different qualities of energy depending on our nature, circumstances, and the work we need to do at a given moment.

In the hands, every finger has a different quality. The small finger is in relation with the earth element, the ring finger with water, the middle finger with fire, the index with air and the thumb with ether. Knowledge of this can help us to an extent.

The parts of the body are in direct relation to the emotions and the functions of the brain. Each of them has a different kind of energy. If the different qualities of the five elements influence our bodies, it is important to know how we can use them to our advantage.

The positioning of the fingers and hands, is called a *mudra*. A *mudra* has a different effect on us depending on how we use our fingers. A *mudra* is a special posture where the fingers and hands produce a different kind of feeling and experience on our energy level, body and mind.

This is also in direct relation to reiki postures, because a different effect is produced depending on where we put our hands.

In a therapy session, the hand can be placed anywhere the patient feels comfortable but in kinesic techniques are used information from the brain. therapy sessions it was accidentally discovered, by observing the behaviour of muscles depending on the place the patient was touched, that our hand can affect the movement of energy. When a very specific work, like in kinesiology, is done, it is necessary to have a lot of control. But when the work is based on a more spontaneous movement of energy, similar to reiki, so much control is not necessary. This is because the body relates with the brain and functions can be stimulated with the contact of the hand. Finger possibilities are more specific. In kinesiology, special kinds of *mudras* are used, which are made by the therapist and patient, as codes to connect with the brain and energy for information.

There are different postures in meditation of which some affect the electrical functions, and the others emotional, chemical or structural functions. The energy of the five elements affect us, depending on our posture. We can produce the effect we want by consciously combining touch between selected fingertips. Sometimes it is necessary that our nails touch a particular superior part at the border o. the three different parts (two a. thumb), between the articulation (knuckles) of the fingers. We can also open our hands into different postures as in drawings of Indian gods or goddesses.

We can put our hands together in an attitude of prayer, to connect our male and female parts and close our energy circle, offering ourselves to God.

It is also beneficial to practise rythmic movements with the hands and fingers.

It is natural to do this to the sound of music, and in some dances, particularly oriental dances. Many things can be expressed with the hands, and lots of energy can be moved. Everything we do with our hands should be pure. Develop the practice of paying attention while doing things with your hands, i.e. writing. Do it lovingly and enjoy it. The therapy will be helpful.

We should put a loving energy into all our acts, and to feel the divine energy flowing through them. Every action must be done consciously, concentrating completely on what we are doing, and offering it back to the fountain of divine love.

Conclusion

In conclusion, I would like to emphasise that it is not anybody who heals anybody else. The techniques to work on pressure points are mastered by some who are able to help others to effect the vital energy to be in balance, which helps to heal patients. The mind is the most important factor. The mind is very powerful and can become balanced or imbalanced.

Positive thoughts are important, negative thoughts can produce a new imbalance.

I believe that faith and trust are very important. They must be the only feelings (thoughts) in our minds. Faith forcefully moves energy towards healing.

When a person thinks positively, having a strong will power, all the energy, from every part of his being, becomes focused on the goal and he succeeds, in spite of the alarmingly negative situation.

Thus, the power of our mind is very strong and to use it in a positive way is to use the power of love, which is the greatest of any power in creation.